How to use this food journal:

This is meant to be a guide, not a rule. Use it as you see fit, do what you want. Fuck the system.

Ideally, you'll record your meals and snacks, as well as how you felt after you ate. Make a note of your movement, water, energy, and sleep. If you take supplements, record that too.

At the end of the day, take some time to write out 3 things you're grateful for. Studies show that a 5-minute gratitude practice can increase happiness, deepen relationships, improve work performance and boost energy as well as the immune system.

When your week is done, check in with yourself. What went well? What could have gone better? And what's a managable goal for next week (be honest with yourself, you're not gonna suddenly run a marathon or drop 20 lbs in a week. What's a helpful step towards your big goal?)

At the end of the month, take it a step further and do some self-evaluation. Is there a pattern in your diet and mood? Or your energy and water intake? Knowledge is power, and with more info about your individual body you can make the best choices for you!

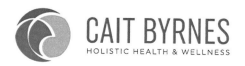

CAIT BYRNES
HOLISTIC HEALTH & WELLNESS

Today is:____ / ____ / ____

Breakfast:_____   I felt:_____
_____   _____

Snack:_____   I felt:_____
_____   _____

Lunch:_____   I felt:_____
_____   _____

Snack:_____   I felt:_____
_____   _____

Dinner:_____   I felt:_____
_____   _____

Snack:_____   I felt:_____
_____   _____

Glasses of water (8oz) :_____

Other Beverages:_____

Movement for today:_____

Did you take your supplements?   Damn right   I forgot

How was your sleep last night?_____

What was your energy level today? Low   Eh   Pretty Good   Fan-fucking-tastic!

Today I'm grateful for:

1._____

2._____

3._____

Today is:___ /___ /___

Breakfast:_____   I felt:_____
_____   _____

Snack:_____   I felt:_____
_____   _____

Lunch:_____   I felt:_____
_____   _____

Snack:_____   I felt:_____
_____   _____

Dinner:_____   I felt:_____
_____   _____

Snack:_____   I felt:_____
_____   _____

Glasses of water (8oz) :_____

Other Beverages:_____

Movement for today:_____

Did you take your supplements?   Damn right   I forgot

How was your sleep last night?_____

What was your energy level today? Low   Eh   Pretty Good   Fan-fucking-tastic!

Today I'm grateful for:

1._____

2._____

3._____

Today is:___ /___ /___

Breakfast:_____ | I felt:_____
_____ | _____

Snack:_____ | I felt:_____
_____ | _____

Lunch:_____ | I felt:_____
_____ | _____

Snack:_____ | I felt:_____
_____ | _____

Dinner:_____ | I felt:_____
_____ | _____

Snack:_____ | I felt:_____
_____ | _____

Glasses of water (8oz) :_____

Other Beverages:_____

Movement for today:_____

Did you take your supplements?   Damn right   I forgot

How was your sleep last night?_____

What was your energy level today?   Low   Eh   Pretty Good   Fan-fucking-tastic!

Today I'm grateful for:

1._____

2._____

3._____

Today is:____ /____ /____

Breakfast:_____   I felt:_____

_____   _____

Snack:_____   I felt:_____

_____   _____

Lunch:_____   I felt:_____

_____   _____

Snack:_____   I felt:_____

_____   _____

Dinner:_____   I felt:_____

_____   _____

Snack:_____   I felt:_____

_____   _____

Glasses of water (8oz) :_____

Other Beverages:_____

Movement for today:_____

Did you take your supplements?   Damn right   I forgot

How was your sleep last night?_____

What was your energy level today?   Low   Eh   Pretty Good   Fan-fucking-tastic!

Today I'm grateful for:

1._____

2._____

3._____

Today is:___ /___ /___

Breakfast:_____   I felt:_____
_____   _____

Snack:_____   I felt:_____
_____   _____

Lunch:_____   I felt:_____
_____   _____

Snack:_____   I felt:_____
_____   _____

Dinner:_____   I felt:_____
_____   _____

Snack:_____   I felt:_____
_____   _____

Glasses of water (8oz) :_____

Other Beverages:_____

Movement for today:_____

Did you take your supplements?   Damn right   I forgot

How was your sleep last night?_____

What was your energy level today?   Low   Eh   Pretty Good   Fan-fucking-tastic!

Today I'm grateful for:

1._____

2._____

3._____

Today is:___ /___ /___

Breakfast:_____   I felt:_____
_____   _____

Snack:_____   I felt:_____
_____   _____

Lunch:_____   I felt:_____
_____   _____

Snack:_____   I felt:_____
_____   _____

Dinner:_____   I felt:_____
_____   _____

Snack:_____   I felt:_____
_____   _____

Glasses of water (8oz) :_____

Other Beverages:_____

Movement for today:_____

Did you take your supplements?   Damn right   I forgot

How was your sleep last night?_____

What was your energy level today?   Low   Eh   Pretty Good   Fan-fucking-tastic!

Today I'm grateful for:

1._____

2._____

3._____

Today is:_____ /_____ /_____

Breakfast:_____   I felt:_____

_____   _____

Snack:_____   I felt:_____

_____   _____

Lunch:_____   I felt:_____

_____   _____

Snack:_____   I felt:_____

_____   _____

Dinner:_____   I felt:_____

_____   _____

Snack:_____   I felt:_____

_____   _____

Glasses of water (8oz) :_____

Other Beverages:_____

Movement for today:_____

Did you take your supplements?   Damn right   I forgot

How was your sleep last night?_____

What was your energy level today?   Low   Eh   Pretty Good   Fan-fucking-tastic!

Today I'm grateful for:

1._____

2._____

3._____

Check in, Yo

In general, this week I felt:_____

_____

_____

_____

_____

My self-care practice included:_____

_____

_____

_____

_____

These decisions did not support me:_____

_____

_____

_____

_____

Next week, my goal is:_____

_____

_____

_____

_____

Today is:___ /___ /___

Breakfast:_____   I felt:_____

_____   _____

Snack:_____   I felt:_____

_____   _____

Lunch:_____   I felt:_____

_____   _____

Snack:_____   I felt:_____

_____   _____

Dinner:_____   I felt:_____

_____   _____

Snack:_____   I felt:_____

_____   _____

Glasses of water (8oz) :_____

Other Beverages:_____

Movement for today:_____

Did you take your supplements?   Damn right   I forgot

How was your sleep last night?_____

What was your energy level today?   Low   Eh   Pretty Good   Fan-fucking-tastic!

Today I'm grateful for:

1._____

2._____

3._____

Today is:___ /___ /___

Breakfast:_____   I felt:_____

_____   _____

Snack:_____   I felt:_____

_____   _____

Lunch:_____   I felt:_____

_____   _____

Snack:_____   I felt:_____

_____   _____

Dinner:_____   I felt:_____

_____   _____

Snack:_____   I felt:_____

_____   _____

Glasses of water (8oz) :_____

Other Beverages:_____

Movement for today:_____

Did you take your supplements?   Damn right   I forgot

How was your sleep last night?_____

What was your energy level today?   Low   Eh   Pretty Good   Fan-fucking-tastic!

Today I'm grateful for:

1._____

2._____

3._____

Today is:___ /___ /___

Breakfast:_____   I felt:_____
_____   _____

Snack:_____   I felt:_____
_____   _____

Lunch:_____   I felt:_____
_____   _____

Snack:_____   I felt:_____
_____   _____

Dinner:_____   I felt:_____
_____   _____

Snack:_____   I felt:_____
_____   _____

Glasses of water (8oz) :_____

Other Beverages:_____

Movement for today:_____

Did you take your supplements?   Damn right   I forgot

How was your sleep last night?_____

What was your energy level today?   Low   Eh   Pretty Good   Fan-fucking-tastic!

Today I'm grateful for:

1._____

2._____

3._____

Today is:___ /___ /___

Breakfast:_____   I felt:_____
_____   _____

Snack:_____   I felt:_____
_____   _____

Lunch:_____   I felt:_____
_____   _____

Snack:_____   I felt:_____
_____   _____

Dinner:_____   I felt:_____
_____   _____

Snack:_____   I felt:_____
_____   _____

Glasses of water (8oz) :_____

Other Beverages:_____

Movement for today:_____

Did you take your supplements?   Damn right   I forgot

How was your sleep last night?_____

What was your energy level today?   Low   Eh   Pretty Good   Fan-fucking-tastic!

Today I'm grateful for:

1._____
2._____
3._____

Today is:____ /____ /____

Breakfast:_____ I felt:_____
_____ _____

Snack:_____ I felt:_____
_____ _____

Lunch:_____ I felt:_____
_____ _____

Snack:_____ I felt:_____
_____ _____

Dinner:_____ I felt:_____
_____ _____

Snack:_____ I felt:_____
_____ _____

Glasses of water (8oz) :_____

Other Beverages:_____

Movement for today:_____

Did you take your supplements?   Damn right   I forgot

How was your sleep last night?_____

What was your energy level today?   Low   Eh   Pretty Good   Fan-fucking-tastic!

Today I'm grateful for:

1._____

2._____

3._____

Today is:____ /____ /____

Breakfast:_____   I felt:_____
_____   _____

Snack:_____   I felt:_____
_____   _____

Lunch:_____   I felt:_____
_____   _____

Snack:_____   I felt:_____
_____   _____

Dinner:_____   I felt:_____
_____   _____

Snack:_____   I felt:_____
_____   _____

Glasses of water (8oz) :_____

Other Beverages:_____

Movement for today:_____

Did you take your supplements?   Damn right   I forgot

How was your sleep last night?_____

What was your energy level today?   Low   Eh   Pretty Good   Fan-fucking-tastic!

Today I'm grateful for:

1._____

2._____

3._____

Today is:____ /____ /____

Breakfast:_____   I felt:_____
_____   _____

Snack:_____   I felt:_____
_____   _____

Lunch:_____   I felt:_____
_____   _____

Snack:_____   I felt:_____
_____   _____

Dinner:_____   I felt:_____
_____   _____

Snack:_____   I felt:_____
_____   _____

Glasses of water (8oz) :_____

Other Beverages:_____

Movement for today:_____

Did you take your supplements?   Damn right   I forgot

How was your sleep last night?_____

What was your energy level today?   Low   Eh   Pretty Good   Fan-fucking-tastic!

Today I'm grateful for:

1._____

2._____

3._____

Check in, Yo

In general, this week I felt:_____

_____

_____

_____

_____

My self-care practice included:_____

_____

_____

_____

_____

These decisions did not support me:_____

_____

_____

_____

_____

Next week, my goal is:_____

_____

_____

_____

_____

Today is:____ /____ /____

Breakfast:_____   I felt:_____

_____   _____

Snack:_____   I felt:_____

_____   _____

Lunch:_____   I felt:_____

_____   _____

Snack:_____   I felt:_____

_____   _____

Dinner:_____   I felt:_____

_____   _____

Snack:_____   I felt:_____

_____   _____

Glasses of water (8oz) :_____

Other Beverages:_____

Movement for today:_____

Did you take your supplements?   Damn right   I forgot

How was your sleep last night?_____

What was your energy level today?   Low   Eh   Pretty Good   Fan-fucking-tastic!

Today I'm grateful for:

1._____

2._____

3._____

Today is:___ /___ /___

Breakfast:_____   I felt:_____
_____   _____

Snack:_____   I felt:_____
_____   _____

Lunch:_____   I felt:_____
_____   _____

Snack:_____   I felt:_____
_____   _____

Dinner:_____   I felt:_____
_____   _____

Snack:_____   I felt:_____
_____   _____

Glasses of water (8oz) :_____

Other Beverages:_____

Movement for today:_____

Did you take your supplements?   Damn right   I forgot

How was your sleep last night?_____

What was your energy level today? Low   Eh   Pretty Good   Fan-fucking-tastic!

Today I'm grateful for:

1._____

2._____

3._____

Today is:___ /___ /___

Breakfast:_____   I felt:_____
_____   _____

Snack:_____   I felt:_____
_____   _____

Lunch:_____   I felt:_____
_____   _____

Snack:_____   I felt:_____
_____   _____

Dinner:_____   I felt:_____
_____   _____

Snack:_____   I felt:_____
_____   _____

Glasses of water (8oz) :_____

Other Beverages:_____

Movement for today:_____

Did you take your supplements?   Damn right   I forgot

How was your sleep last night?_____

What was your energy level today?   Low   Eh   Pretty Good   Fan-fucking-tastic!

Today I'm grateful for:

1._____

2._____

3._____

Today is:___ /___ /___

Breakfast:_____   I felt:_____
_____   _____

Snack:_____   I felt:_____
_____   _____

Lunch:_____   I felt:_____
_____   _____

Snack:_____   I felt:_____
_____   _____

Dinner:_____   I felt:_____
_____   _____

Snack:_____   I felt:_____
_____   _____

Glasses of water (8oz) :_____

Other Beverages:_____

Movement for today:_____

Did you take your supplements?   Damn right   I forgot

How was your sleep last night?_____

What was your energy level today?   Low   Eh   Pretty Good   Fan-fucking-tastic!

Today I'm grateful for:

1._____

2._____

3._____

Today is:___ /___ /___

Breakfast:_____   I felt:_____

_____   _____

Snack:_____   I felt:_____

_____   _____

Lunch:_____   I felt:_____

_____   _____

Snack:_____   I felt:_____

_____   _____

Dinner:_____   I felt:_____

_____   _____

Snack:_____   I felt:_____

_____   _____

Glasses of water (8oz) :_____

Other Beverages:_____

Movement for today:_____

Did you take your supplements?   Damn right   I forgot

How was your sleep last night?_____

What was your energy level today?   Low   Eh   Pretty Good   Fan-fucking-tastic!

Today I'm grateful for:

1._____

2._____

3._____

Today is:_____ /_____ /_____

Breakfast:_____   I felt:_____
_____   _____

Snack:_____   I felt:_____
_____   _____

Lunch:_____   I felt:_____
_____   _____

Snack:_____   I felt:_____
_____   _____

Dinner:_____   I felt:_____
_____   _____

Snack:_____   I felt:_____
_____   _____

Glasses of water (8oz) :_____

Other Beverages:_____

Movement for today:_____

Did you take your supplements?   Damn right   I forgot

How was your sleep last night?_____

What was your energy level today?   Low   Eh   Pretty Good   Fan-fucking-tastic!

Today I'm grateful for:

1._____

2._____

3._____

Today is:___ /___ /___

Breakfast:_____   I felt:_____
_____   _____

Snack:_____   I felt:_____
_____   _____

Lunch:_____   I felt:_____
_____   _____

Snack:_____   I felt:_____
_____   _____

Dinner:_____   I felt:_____
_____   _____

Snack:_____   I felt:_____
_____   _____

Glasses of water (8oz) :_____

Other Beverages:_____

Movement for today:_____

Did you take your supplements?   Damn right   I forgot

How was your sleep last night?_____

What was your energy level today?   Low   Eh   Pretty Good   Fan-fucking-tastic!

Today I'm grateful for:

1._____

2._____

3._____

Check in, Yo

In general, this week I felt:_____

_____

_____

_____

_____

My self-care practice included:_____

_____

_____

_____

_____

These decisions did not support me:_____

_____

_____

_____

_____

Next week, my goal is:_____

_____

_____

_____

_____

Today is:____ /____ /____

Breakfast:_____   I felt:_____
_____   _____

Snack:_____   I felt:_____
_____   _____

Lunch:_____   I felt:_____
_____   _____

Snack:_____   I felt:_____
_____   _____

Dinner:_____   I felt:_____
_____   _____

Snack:_____   I felt:_____
_____   _____

Glasses of water (8oz) :_____

Other Beverages:_____

Movement for today:_____

Did you take your supplements?   Damn right   I forgot

How was your sleep last night?_____

What was your energy level today?   Low   Eh   Pretty Good   Fan-fucking-tastic!

Today I'm grateful for:

1._____

2._____

3._____

Today is:____ /____ /____

Breakfast:_____   I felt:_____

_____   _____

Snack:_____   I felt:_____

_____   _____

Lunch:_____   I felt:_____

_____   _____

Snack:_____   I felt:_____

_____   _____

Dinner:_____   I felt:_____

_____   _____

Snack:_____   I felt:_____

_____   _____

Glasses of water (8oz) :_____

Other Beverages:_____

Movement for today:_____

Did you take your supplements?   Damn right   I forgot

How was your sleep last night?_____

What was your energy level today?   Low   Eh   Pretty Good   Fan-fucking-tastic!

Today I'm grateful for:

1._____

2._____

3._____

Today is:____ /____ /____

Breakfast:_____ I felt:_____

_____ _____

Snack:_____ I felt:_____

_____ _____

Lunch:_____ I felt:_____

_____ _____

Snack:_____ I felt:_____

_____ _____

Dinner:_____ I felt:_____

_____ _____

Snack:_____ I felt:_____

_____ _____

Glasses of water (8oz) :_____

Other Beverages:_____

Movement for today:_____

Did you take your supplements?   Damn right   I forgot

How was your sleep last night?_____

What was your energy level today?   Low   Eh   Pretty Good   Fan-fucking-tastic!

Today I'm grateful for:

1._____

2._____

3._____

Today is:____ /____ /____

Breakfast:_____   I felt:_____
_____   _____

Snack:_____   I felt:_____
_____   _____

Lunch:_____   I felt:_____
_____   _____

Snack:_____   I felt:_____
_____   _____

Dinner:_____   I felt:_____
_____   _____

Snack:_____   I felt:_____
_____   _____

Glasses of water (8oz) :_____

Other Beverages:_____

Movement for today:_____

Did you take your supplements?   Damn right   I forgot

How was your sleep last night?_____

What was your energy level today?   Low   Eh   Pretty Good   Fan-fucking-tastic!

Today I'm grateful for:

1._____

2._____

3._____

Today is:___ /___ /___

Breakfast:_____   I felt:_____

_____   _____

Snack:_____   I felt:_____

_____   _____

Lunch:_____   I felt:_____

_____   _____

Snack:_____   I felt:_____

_____   _____

Dinner:_____   I felt:_____

_____   _____

Snack:_____   I felt:_____

_____   _____

Glasses of water (8oz) :_____

Other Beverages:_____

Movement for today:_____

Did you take your supplements?   Damn right   I forgot

How was your sleep last night?_____

What was your energy level today?   Low   Eh   Pretty Good   Fan-fucking-tastic!

Today I'm grateful for:

1._____

2._____

3._____

Today is:_____ /_____ /_____

Breakfast:_____   I felt:_____

_____   _____

Snack:_____   I felt:_____

_____   _____

Lunch:_____   I felt:_____

_____   _____

Snack:_____   I felt:_____

_____   _____

Dinner:_____   I felt:_____

_____   _____

Snack:_____   I felt:_____

_____   _____

Glasses of water (8oz) :_____

Other Beverages:_____

Movement for today:_____

Did you take your supplements?   Damn right   I forgot

How was your sleep last night?_____

What was your energy level today?   Low   Eh   Pretty Good   Fan-fucking-tastic!

Today I'm grateful for:

1._____

2._____

3._____

Today is:___ /___ /___

Breakfast:_____   I felt:_____

_____   _____

Snack:_____   I felt:_____

_____   _____

Lunch:_____   I felt:_____

_____   _____

Snack:_____   I felt:_____

_____   _____

Dinner:_____   I felt:_____

_____   _____

Snack:_____   I felt:_____

_____   _____

Glasses of water (8oz) :_____

Other Beverages:_____

Movement for today:_____

Did you take your supplements?   Damn right   I forgot

How was your sleep last night?_____

What was your energy level today?   Low   Eh   Pretty Good   Fan-fucking-tastic!

Today I'm grateful for:

1._____

2._____

3._____

Check in, Yo

In general, this week I felt:_____

_____

_____

_____

_____

My self-care practice included:_____

_____

_____

_____

_____

These decisions did not support me:_____

_____

_____

_____

_____

Next week, my goal is:_____

_____

_____

_____

_____

How'd It Go?

Go back through the past month. Do you notice any patterns in your food and mood?

Example: "I felt more tired when I didn't drink water."

"I was happier on days I ate snacks"

"I had more energy when I brought lunch to work"

_____

_____

_____

_____

What are you gonna do about it?

_____

_____

_____

_____

List some awesome things that happened this month:

_____

_____

_____

_____

you're the fucking best

Today is:___ /___ /___

Breakfast:_____   I felt:_____
_____   _____

Snack:_____   I felt:_____
_____   _____

Lunch:_____   I felt:_____
_____   _____

Snack:_____   I felt:_____
_____   _____

Dinner:_____   I felt:_____
_____   _____

Snack:_____   I felt:_____
_____   _____

Glasses of water (8oz) :_____

Other Beverages:_____

Movement for today:_____

Did you take your supplements?   Damn right   I forgot

How was your sleep last night?_____

What was your energy level today?   Low   Eh   Pretty Good   Fan-fucking-tastic!

Today I'm grateful for:

1._____

2._____

3._____

Today is:___ /___ /___

Breakfast:_____   I felt:_____
_____   _____

Snack:_____   I felt:_____
_____   _____

Lunch:_____   I felt:_____
_____   _____

Snack:_____   I felt:_____
_____   _____

Dinner:_____   I felt:_____
_____   _____

Snack:_____   I felt:_____
_____   _____

Glasses of water (8oz) :_____

Other Beverages:_____

Movement for today:_____

Did you take your supplements?   Damn right   I forgot

How was your sleep last night?_____

What was your energy level today?   Low   Eh   Pretty Good   Fan-fucking-tastic!

Today I'm grateful for:

1._____

2._____

3._____

Today is:___ /___ /___

Breakfast:_____   I felt:_____
_____   _____

Snack:_____   I felt:_____
_____   _____

Lunch:_____   I felt:_____
_____   _____

Snack:_____   I felt:_____
_____   _____

Dinner:_____   I felt:_____
_____   _____

Snack:_____   I felt:_____
_____   _____

Glasses of water (8oz) :_____

Other Beverages:_____

Movement for today:_____

Did you take your supplements?   Damn right   I forgot

How was your sleep last night?_____

What was your energy level today?   Low   Eh   Pretty Good   Fan-fucking-tastic!

Today I'm grateful for:

1._____

2._____

3._____

Today is:____ /____ /____

Breakfast:_____   I felt:_____
_____   _____

Snack:_____   I felt:_____
_____   _____

Lunch:_____   I felt:_____
_____   _____

Snack:_____   I felt:_____
_____   _____

Dinner:_____   I felt:_____
_____   _____

Snack:_____   I felt:_____
_____   _____

Glasses of water (8oz) :_____

Other Beverages:_____

Movement for today:_____

Did you take your supplements?   Damn right   I forgot

How was your sleep last night?_____

What was your energy level today?   Low   Eh   Pretty Good   Fan-fucking-tastic!

Today I'm grateful for:

1._____

2._____

3._____

Today is:____ /____ /____

Breakfast:_____   I felt:_____
_____   _____

Snack:_____   I felt:_____
_____   _____

Lunch:_____   I felt:_____
_____   _____

Snack:_____   I felt:_____
_____   _____

Dinner:_____   I felt:_____
_____   _____

Snack:_____   I felt:_____
_____   _____

Glasses of water (8oz) :_____

Other Beverages:_____

Movement for today:_____

Did you take your supplements?   Damn right   I forgot

How was your sleep last night?_____

What was your energy level today?   Low   Eh   Pretty Good   Fan-fucking-tastic!

Today I'm grateful for:

1._____

2._____

3._____

Today is:___ /___ /___

Breakfast:_____   I felt:_____

_____   _____

Snack:_____   I felt:_____

_____   _____

Lunch:_____   I felt:_____

_____   _____

Snack:_____   I felt:_____

_____   _____

Dinner:_____   I felt:_____

_____   _____

Snack:_____   I felt:_____

_____   _____

Glasses of water (8oz) :_____

Other Beverages:_____

Movement for today:_____

Did you take your supplements?   Damn right   I forgot

How was your sleep last night?_____

What was your energy level today?   Low   Eh   Pretty Good   Fan-fucking-tastic!

Today I'm grateful for:

1._____

2._____

3._____

Today is:___ /___ /___

Breakfast:_____   I felt:_____
_____   _____

Snack:_____   I felt:_____
_____   _____

Lunch:_____   I felt:_____
_____   _____

Snack:_____   I felt:_____
_____   _____

Dinner:_____   I felt:_____
_____   _____

Snack:_____   I felt:_____
_____   _____

Glasses of water (8oz) :_____

Other Beverages:_____

Movement for today:_____

Did you take your supplements?   Damn right   I forgot

How was your sleep last night?_____

What was your energy level today?   Low   Eh   Pretty Good   Fan-fucking-tastic!

Today I'm grateful for:

1._____

2._____

3._____

Check in, Yo

In general, this week I felt:_____

_____

_____

_____

_____

My self-care practice included:_____

_____

_____

_____

_____

These decisions did not support me:_____

_____

_____

_____

_____

Next week, my goal is:_____

_____

_____

_____

_____

Today is:____ /____ /____

Breakfast:_____   I felt:_____
_____   _____

Snack:_____   I felt:_____
_____   _____

Lunch:_____   I felt:_____
_____   _____

Snack:_____   I felt:_____
_____   _____

Dinner:_____   I felt:_____
_____   _____

Snack:_____   I felt:_____
_____   _____

Glasses of water (8oz) :_____

Other Beverages:_____

Movement for today:_____

Did you take your supplements?   Damn right   I forgot

How was your sleep last night?_____

What was your energy level today?   Low   Eh   Pretty Good   Fan-fucking-tastic!

Today I'm grateful for:

1._____

2._____

3._____

Today is:___ /___ /___

Breakfast:_____

_____

I felt:_____

_____

Snack:_____

_____

I felt:_____

_____

Lunch:_____

_____

I felt:_____

_____

Snack:_____

_____

I felt:_____

_____

Dinner:_____

_____

I felt:_____

_____

Snack:_____

_____

I felt:_____

_____

Glasses of water (8oz) :_____

Other Beverages:_____

Movement for today:_____

Did you take your supplements?   Damn right   I forgot

How was your sleep last night?_____

What was your energy level today?   Low   Eh   Pretty Good   Fan-fucking-tastic!

Today I'm grateful for:

1._____

2._____

3._____

Today is:___ /___ /___

Breakfast:_____ | I felt:_____
_____ | _____

Snack:_____ | I felt:_____
_____ | _____

Lunch:_____ | I felt:_____
_____ | _____

Snack:_____ | I felt:_____
_____ | _____

Dinner:_____ | I felt:_____
_____ | _____

Snack:_____ | I felt:_____
_____ | _____

Glasses of water (8oz) :_____

Other Beverages:_____

Movement for today:_____

Did you take your supplements?   Damn right   I forgot

How was your sleep last night?_____

What was your energy level today?   Low   Eh   Pretty Good   Fan-fucking-tastic!

Today I'm grateful for:

1._____

2._____

3._____

Today is:_____ /_____ /_____

Breakfast:_____   I felt:_____

_____   _____

Snack:_____   I felt:_____

_____   _____

Lunch:_____   I felt:_____

_____   _____

Snack:_____   I felt:_____

_____   _____

Dinner:_____   I felt:_____

_____   _____

Snack:_____   I felt:_____

_____   _____

Glasses of water (8oz) :_____

Other Beverages:_____

Movement for today:_____

Did you take your supplements?   Damn right   I forgot

How was your sleep last night?_____

What was your energy level today?   Low   Eh   Pretty Good   Fan-fucking-tastic!

Today I'm grateful for:

1._____

2._____

3._____

Today is:____ /____ /____

Breakfast:_____   I felt:_____
_____   _____

Snack:_____   I felt:_____
_____   _____

Lunch:_____   I felt:_____
_____   _____

Snack:_____   I felt:_____
_____   _____

Dinner:_____   I felt:_____
_____   _____

Snack:_____   I felt:_____
_____   _____

Glasses of water (8oz) :_____

Other Beverages:_____

Movement for today:_____

Did you take your supplements?   Damn right   I forgot

How was your sleep last night?_____

What was your energy level today?   Low   Eh   Pretty Good   Fan-fucking-tastic!

Today I'm grateful for:

1._____

2._____

3._____

Today is:___ /___ /___

Breakfast:_____   I felt:_____

_____   _____

Snack:_____   I felt:_____

_____   _____

Lunch:_____   I felt:_____

_____   _____

Snack:_____   I felt:_____

_____   _____

Dinner:_____   I felt:_____

_____   _____

Snack:_____   I felt:_____

_____   _____

Glasses of water (8oz) :_____

Other Beverages:_____

Movement for today:_____

Did you take your supplements?   Damn right   I forgot

How was your sleep last night?_____

What was your energy level today? Low   Eh   Pretty Good   Fan-fucking-tastic!

Today I'm grateful for:

1._____

2._____

3._____

Today is:____ /____ /____

Breakfast:_____   I felt:_____
_____   _____

Snack:_____   I felt:_____
_____   _____

Lunch:_____   I felt:_____
_____   _____

Snack:_____   I felt:_____
_____   _____

Dinner:_____   I felt:_____
_____   _____

Snack:_____   I felt:_____
_____   _____

Glasses of water (8oz) :_____

Other Beverages:_____

Movement for today:_____

Did you take your supplements?   Damn right   I forgot

How was your sleep last night?_____

What was your energy level today?   Low   Eh   Pretty Good   Fan-fucking-tastic!

Today I'm grateful for:

1._____

2._____

3._____

Check in, Yo

In general, this week I felt:_____

_____

_____

_____

_____

My self-care practice included:_____

_____

_____

_____

_____

These decisions did not support me:_____

_____

_____

_____

_____

Next week, my goal is:_____

_____

_____

_____

_____

Today is:___ /___ /___

Breakfast:_____   I felt:_____

_____   _____

Snack:_____   I felt:_____

_____   _____

Lunch:_____   I felt:_____

_____   _____

Snack:_____   I felt:_____

_____   _____

Dinner:_____   I felt:_____

_____   _____

Snack:_____   I felt:_____

_____   _____

Glasses of water (8oz) :_____

Other Beverages:_____

Movement for today:_____

Did you take your supplements?   Damn right   I forgot

How was your sleep last night?_____

What was your energy level today?   Low   Eh   Pretty Good   Fan-fucking-tastic!

Today I'm grateful for:

1._____

2._____

3._____

Today is:____ /____ /____

Breakfast:_____   I felt:_____

_____   _____

Snack:_____   I felt:_____

_____   _____

Lunch:_____   I felt:_____

_____   _____

Snack:_____   I felt:_____

_____   _____

Dinner:_____   I felt:_____

_____   _____

Snack:_____   I felt:_____

_____   _____

Glasses of water (8oz) :_____

Other Beverages:_____

Movement for today:_____

Did you take your supplements?   Damn right   I forgot

How was your sleep last night?_____

What was your energy level today?   Low   Eh   Pretty Good   Fan-fucking-tastic!

Today I'm grateful for:

1._____

2._____

3._____

Today is:___ /___ /___

Breakfast:_____   I felt:_____

_____   _____

Snack:_____   I felt:_____

_____   _____

Lunch:_____   I felt:_____

_____   _____

Snack:_____   I felt:_____

_____   _____

Dinner:_____   I felt:_____

_____   _____

Snack:_____   I felt:_____

_____   _____

Glasses of water (8oz) :_____

Other Beverages:_____

Movement for today:_____

Did you take your supplements?   Damn right   I forgot

How was your sleep last night?_____

What was your energy level today?   Low   Eh   Pretty Good   Fan-fucking-tastic!

Today I'm grateful for:

1._____

2._____

3._____

Today is:___ /___ /___

Breakfast:_____   I felt:_____

_____   _____

Snack:_____   I felt:_____

_____   _____

Lunch:_____   I felt:_____

_____   _____

Snack:_____   I felt:_____

_____   _____

Dinner:_____   I felt:_____

_____   _____

Snack:_____   I felt:_____

_____   _____

Glasses of water (8oz) :_____

Other Beverages:_____

Movement for today:_____

Did you take your supplements?   Damn right   I forgot

How was your sleep last night?_____

What was your energy level today?   Low   Eh   Pretty Good   Fan-fucking-tastic!

Today I'm grateful for:

1._____

2._____

3._____

Today is:____ /____ /____

Breakfast:_____   I felt:_____

_____   _____

Snack:_____   I felt:_____

_____   _____

Lunch:_____   I felt:_____

_____   _____

Snack:_____   I felt:_____

_____   _____

Dinner:_____   I felt:_____

_____   _____

Snack:_____   I felt:_____

_____   _____

Glasses of water (8oz) :_____

Other Beverages:_____

Movement for today:_____

Did you take your supplements?   Damn right   I forgot

How was your sleep last night?_____

What was your energy level today?   Low   Eh   Pretty Good   Fan-fucking-tastic!

Today I'm grateful for:

1._____

2._____

3._____

Today is:___ /___ /___

Breakfast:_____   I felt:_____

_____   _____

Snack:_____   I felt:_____

_____   _____

Lunch:_____   I felt:_____

_____   _____

Snack:_____   I felt:_____

_____   _____

Dinner:_____   I felt:_____

_____   _____

Snack:_____   I felt:_____

_____   _____

Glasses of water (8oz) :_____

Other Beverages:_____

Movement for today:_____

Did you take your supplements?   Damn right   I forgot

How was your sleep last night?_____

What was your energy level today?   Low   Eh   Pretty Good   Fan-fucking-tastic!

Today I'm grateful for:

1._____

2._____

3._____

Today is:____ /____ /____

Breakfast:_____   I felt:_____
_____   _____

Snack:_____   I felt:_____
_____   _____

Lunch:_____   I felt:_____
_____   _____

Snack:_____   I felt:_____
_____   _____

Dinner:_____   I felt:_____
_____   _____

Snack:_____   I felt:_____
_____   _____

Glasses of water (8oz) :_____

Other Beverages:_____

Movement for today:_____

Did you take your supplements?   Damn right   I forgot

How was your sleep last night?_____

What was your energy level today?   Low   Eh   Pretty Good   Fan-fucking-tastic!

Today I'm grateful for:

1._____

2._____

3._____

Check in, Yo

In general, this week I felt:_____

_____

_____

_____

_____

My self-care practice included:_____

_____

_____

_____

_____

These decisions did not support me:_____

_____

_____

_____

_____

Next week, my goal is:_____

_____

_____

_____

_____

Today is:____ / ____ / ____

Breakfast:_____   I felt:_____

_____   _____

Snack:_____   I felt:_____

_____   _____

Lunch:_____   I felt:_____

_____   _____

Snack:_____   I felt:_____

_____   _____

Dinner:_____   I felt:_____

_____   _____

Snack:_____   I felt:_____

_____   _____

Glasses of water (8oz) :_____

Other Beverages:_____

Movement for today:_____

Did you take your supplements?   Damn right   I forgot

How was your sleep last night?_____

What was your energy level today?   Low   Eh   Pretty Good   Fan-fucking-tastic!

Today I'm grateful for:

1._____

2._____

3._____

Today is:___ /___ /___

Breakfast:_____   I felt:_____
_____   _____

Snack:_____   I felt:_____
_____   _____

Lunch:_____   I felt:_____
_____   _____

Snack:_____   I felt:_____
_____   _____

Dinner:_____   I felt:_____
_____   _____

Snack:_____   I felt:_____
_____   _____

Glasses of water (8oz) :_____

Other Beverages:_____

Movement for today:_____

Did you take your supplements?   Damn right   I forgot

How was your sleep last night?_____

What was your energy level today? Low Eh Pretty Good Fan-fucking-tastic!

Today I'm grateful for:

1._____

2._____

3._____

Today is:___ /___ /___

Breakfast:_____   I felt:_____
_____   _____

Snack:_____   I felt:_____
_____   _____

Lunch:_____   I felt:_____
_____   _____

Snack:_____   I felt:_____
_____   _____

Dinner:_____   I felt:_____
_____   _____

Snack:_____   I felt:_____
_____   _____

Glasses of water (8oz) :_____

Other Beverages:_____

Movement for today:_____

Did you take your supplements?   Damn right   I forgot

How was your sleep last night?_____

What was your energy level today?   Low   Eh   Pretty Good   Fan-fucking-tastic!

Today I'm grateful for:

1._____

2._____

3._____

Today is:___ /___ /___

Breakfast:_____   I felt:_____

_____   _____

Snack:_____   I felt:_____

_____   _____

Lunch:_____   I felt:_____

_____   _____

Snack:_____   I felt:_____

_____   _____

Dinner:_____   I felt:_____

_____   _____

Snack:_____   I felt:_____

_____   _____

Glasses of water (8oz) :_____

Other Beverages:_____

Movement for today:_____

Did you take your supplements?   Damn right   I forgot

How was your sleep last night?_____

What was your energy level today?   Low   Eh   Pretty Good   Fan-fucking-tastic!

Today I'm grateful for:

1._____

2._____

3._____

Today is:____ /____ /____

Breakfast:_____   I felt:_____
_____   _____

Snack:_____   I felt:_____
_____   _____

Lunch:_____   I felt:_____
_____   _____

Snack:_____   I felt:_____
_____   _____

Dinner:_____   I felt:_____
_____   _____

Snack:_____   I felt:_____
_____   _____

Glasses of water (8oz) :_____

Other Beverages:_____

Movement for today:_____

Did you take your supplements?   Damn right   I forgot

How was your sleep last night?_____

What was your energy level today?   Low   Eh   Pretty Good   Fan-fucking-tastic!

Today I'm grateful for:

1._____

2._____

3._____

Today is:___ /___ /___

Breakfast:_____   I felt:_____

_____   _____

Snack:_____   I felt:_____

_____   _____

Lunch:_____   I felt:_____

_____   _____

Snack:_____   I felt:_____

_____   _____

Dinner:_____   I felt:_____

_____   _____

Snack:_____   I felt:_____

_____   _____

Glasses of water (8oz) :_____

Other Beverages:_____

Movement for today:_____

Did you take your supplements?   Damn right   I forgot

How was your sleep last night?_____

What was your energy level today?   Low   Eh   Pretty Good   Fan-fucking-tastic!

Today I'm grateful for:

1._____

2._____

3._____

Today is:_____ /_____ /_____

Breakfast:_____ I felt:_____
_____ _____

Snack:_____ I felt:_____
_____ _____

Lunch:_____ I felt:_____
_____ _____

Snack:_____ I felt:_____
_____ _____

Dinner:_____ I felt:_____
_____ _____

Snack:_____ I felt:_____
_____ _____

Glasses of water (8oz) :_____
Other Beverages:_____
Movement for today:_____
Did you take your supplements?   Damn right   I forgot
How was your sleep last night?_____
What was your energy level today?   Low   Eh   Pretty Good   Fan-fucking-tastic!

Today I'm grateful for:

1._____
2._____
3._____

Check in, Yo

In general, this week I felt:_____
_____
_____
_____
_____

My self-care practice included:_____
_____
_____
_____
_____

These decisions did not support me:_____
_____
_____
_____
_____

Next week, my goal is:_____
_____
_____
_____
_____

How'd It Go?

Go back through the past month. Do you notice any patterns in your food and mood?

Example: "I felt more tired when I didn't drink water."

"I was happier on days I ate snacks"

"I had more energy when I brought lunch to work"

_____

_____

_____

_____

What are you gonna do about it?

_____

_____

_____

_____

List some awesome things that happened this month:

_____

_____

_____

_____

you're so damn powerful

Today is:___ /___ /___

Breakfast:_____   I felt:_____

_____   _____

Snack:_____   I felt:_____

_____   _____

Lunch:_____   I felt:_____

_____   _____

Snack:_____   I felt:_____

_____   _____

Dinner:_____   I felt:_____

_____   _____

Snack:_____   I felt:_____

_____   _____

Glasses of water (8oz) :_____

Other Beverages:_____

Movement for today:_____

Did you take your supplements?   Damn right   I forgot

How was your sleep last night?_____

What was your energy level today?   Low   Eh   Pretty Good   Fan-fucking-tastic!

Today I'm grateful for:

1._____

2._____

3._____

Today is:____ /____ /____

Breakfast:_____   I felt:_____

_____   _____

Snack:_____   I felt:_____

_____   _____

Lunch:_____   I felt:_____

_____   _____

Snack:_____   I felt:_____

_____   _____

Dinner:_____   I felt:_____

_____   _____

Snack:_____   I felt:_____

_____   _____

Glasses of water (8oz) :_____

Other Beverages:_____

Movement for today:_____

Did you take your supplements?   Damn right   I forgot

How was your sleep last night?_____

What was your energy level today?   Low   Eh   Pretty Good   Fan-fucking-tastic!

Today I'm grateful for:

1._____

2._____

3._____

Today is:___ /___ /___

Breakfast:_____   I felt:_____
_____   _____

Snack:_____   I felt:_____
_____   _____

Lunch:_____   I felt:_____
_____   _____

Snack:_____   I felt:_____
_____   _____

Dinner:_____   I felt:_____
_____   _____

Snack:_____   I felt:_____
_____   _____

Glasses of water (8oz) :_____

Other Beverages:_____

Movement for today:_____

Did you take your supplements?   Damn right   I forgot

How was your sleep last night?_____

What was your energy level today? Low   Eh   Pretty Good   Fan-fucking-tastic!

Today I'm grateful for:

1._____

2._____

3._____

Today is:____ /____ /____

Breakfast:_____   I felt:_____
_____   _____

Snack:_____   I felt:_____
_____   _____

Lunch:_____   I felt:_____
_____   _____

Snack:_____   I felt:_____
_____   _____

Dinner:_____   I felt:_____
_____   _____

Snack:_____   I felt:_____
_____   _____

Glasses of water (8oz) :_____

Other Beverages:_____

Movement for today:_____

Did you take your supplements?   Damn right   I forgot

How was your sleep last night?_____

What was your energy level today?   Low   Eh   Pretty Good   Fan-fucking-tastic!

Today I'm grateful for:

1._____

2._____

3._____

Today is:___ /___ /___

Breakfast:_____   I felt:_____

_____   _____

Snack:_____   I felt:_____

_____   _____

Lunch:_____   I felt:_____

_____   _____

Snack:_____   I felt:_____

_____   _____

Dinner:_____   I felt:_____

_____   _____

Snack:_____   I felt:_____

_____   _____

Glasses of water (8oz) :_____

Other Beverages:_____

Movement for today:_____

Did you take your supplements?   Damn right   I forgot

How was your sleep last night?_____

What was your energy level today? Low   Eh   Pretty Good   Fan-fucking-tastic!

Today I'm grateful for:

1._____

2._____

3._____

Today is:___ /___ /___

Breakfast:_____   I felt:_____
_____   _____

Snack:_____   I felt:_____
_____   _____

Lunch:_____   I felt:_____
_____   _____

Snack:_____   I felt:_____
_____   _____

Dinner:_____   I felt:_____
_____   _____

Snack:_____   I felt:_____
_____   _____

Glasses of water (8oz) :_____

Other Beverages:_____

Movement for today:_____

Did you take your supplements?   Damn right   I forgot

How was your sleep last night?_____

What was your energy level today?   Low   Eh   Pretty Good   Fan-fucking-tastic!

Today I'm grateful for:

1._____

2._____

3._____

Today is:___ /___ /___

Breakfast:_____   I felt:_____

_____   _____

Snack:_____   I felt:_____

_____   _____

Lunch:_____   I felt:_____

_____   _____

Snack:_____   I felt:_____

_____   _____

Dinner:_____   I felt:_____

_____   _____

Snack:_____   I felt:_____

_____   _____

Glasses of water (8oz) :_____

Other Beverages:_____

Movement for today:_____

Did you take your supplements?   Damn right   I forgot

How was your sleep last night?_____

What was your energy level today?   Low   Eh   Pretty Good   Fan-fucking-tastic!

Today I'm grateful for:

1._____

2._____

3._____

Check in, Yo

In general, this week I felt:_____

_____

_____

_____

_____

My self-care practice included:_____

_____

_____

_____

_____

These decisions did not support me:_____

_____

_____

_____

_____

Next week, my goal is:_____

_____

_____

_____

_____

Today is:___ /___ /___

Breakfast:_____   I felt:_____
_____   _____

Snack:_____   I felt:_____
_____   _____

Lunch:_____   I felt:_____
_____   _____

Snack:_____   I felt:_____
_____   _____

Dinner:_____   I felt:_____
_____   _____

Snack:_____   I felt:_____
_____   _____

Glasses of water (8oz) :_____

Other Beverages:_____

Movement for today:_____

Did you take your supplements?   Damn right   I forgot

How was your sleep last night?_____

What was your energy level today?   Low   Eh   Pretty Good   Fan-fucking-tastic!

Today I'm grateful for:

1._____

2._____

3._____

Today is:____ /____ /____

Breakfast:_____   I felt:_____
_____   _____

Snack:_____   I felt:_____
_____   _____

Lunch:_____   I felt:_____
_____   _____

Snack:_____   I felt:_____
_____   _____

Dinner:_____   I felt:_____
_____   _____

Snack:_____   I felt:_____
_____   _____

Glasses of water (8oz) :_____

Other Beverages:_____

Movement for today:_____

Did you take your supplements?   Damn right   I forgot

How was your sleep last night?_____

What was your energy level today?   Low   Eh   Pretty Good   Fan-fucking-tastic!

Today I'm grateful for:

1._____

2._____

3._____

Today is:___ /___ /___

Breakfast:_____ I felt:_____
_____ _____

Snack:_____ I felt:_____
_____ _____

Lunch:_____ I felt:_____
_____ _____

Snack:_____ I felt:_____
_____ _____

Dinner:_____ I felt:_____
_____ _____

Snack:_____ I felt:_____
_____ _____

Glasses of water (8oz) :_____

Other Beverages:_____

Movement for today:_____

Did you take your supplements?   Damn right   I forgot

How was your sleep last night?_____

What was your energy level today?   Low   Eh   Pretty Good   Fan-fucking-tastic!

Today I'm grateful for:

1._____

2._____

3._____

Today is:____ / ____ / ____

Breakfast:_____   I felt:_____
_____   _____

Snack:_____   I felt:_____
_____   _____

Lunch:_____   I felt:_____
_____   _____

Snack:_____   I felt:_____
_____   _____

Dinner:_____   I felt:_____
_____   _____

Snack:_____   I felt:_____
_____   _____

Glasses of water (8oz) :_____

Other Beverages:_____

Movement for today:_____

Did you take your supplements?   Damn right   I forgot

How was your sleep last night?_____

What was your energy level today?   Low   Eh   Pretty Good   Fan-fucking-tastic!

Today I'm grateful for:

1._____

2._____

3._____

Today is:___ /___ /___

Breakfast:_____   I felt:_____
_____   _____

Snack:_____   I felt:_____
_____   _____

Lunch:_____   I felt:_____
_____   _____

Snack:_____   I felt:_____
_____   _____

Dinner:_____   I felt:_____
_____   _____

Snack:_____   I felt:_____
_____   _____

Glasses of water (8oz) :_____

Other Beverages:_____

Movement for today:_____

Did you take your supplements?   Damn right   I forgot

How was your sleep last night?_____

What was your energy level today? Low   Eh   Pretty Good   Fan-fucking-tastic!

Today I'm grateful for:

1._____
2._____
3._____

Today is:____ /____ /____

Breakfast:_____   I felt:_____

_____   _____

Snack:_____   I felt:_____

_____   _____

Lunch:_____   I felt:_____

_____   _____

Snack:_____   I felt:_____

_____   _____

Dinner:_____   I felt:_____

_____   _____

Snack:_____   I felt:_____

_____   _____

Glasses of water (8oz) :_____

Other Beverages:_____

Movement for today:_____

Did you take your supplements?   Damn right   I forgot

How was your sleep last night?_____

What was your energy level today?   Low   Eh   Pretty Good   Fan-fucking-tastic!

Today I'm grateful for:

1._____

2._____

3._____

Today is:___ /___ /___

Breakfast:_____   I felt:_____
_____   _____

Snack:_____   I felt:_____
_____   _____

Lunch:_____   I felt:_____
_____   _____

Snack:_____   I felt:_____
_____   _____

Dinner:_____   I felt:_____
_____   _____

Snack:_____   I felt:_____
_____   _____

Glasses of water (8oz) :_____

Other Beverages:_____

Movement for today:_____

Did you take your supplements?   Damn right   I forgot

How was your sleep last night?_____

What was your energy level today? Low   Eh   Pretty Good   Fan-fucking-tastic!

Today I'm grateful for:

1._____

2._____

3._____

Check in, Yo

In general, this week I felt:_____
_____
_____
_____
_____

My self-care practice included:_____
_____
_____
_____
_____

These decisions did not support me:_____
_____
_____
_____
_____

Next week, my goal is:_____
_____
_____
_____
_____

Today is:___ /___ /___

Breakfast:_____   I felt:_____
_____   _____

Snack:_____   I felt:_____
_____   _____

Lunch:_____   I felt:_____
_____   _____

Snack:_____   I felt:_____
_____   _____

Dinner:_____   I felt:_____
_____   _____

Snack:_____   I felt:_____
_____   _____

Glasses of water (8oz) :_____

Other Beverages:_____

Movement for today:_____

Did you take your supplements?   Damn right   I forgot

How was your sleep last night?_____

What was your energy level today?   Low   Eh   Pretty Good   Fan-fucking-tastic!

Today I'm grateful for:

1._____

2._____

3._____

Today is:____ /____ /____

Breakfast:_____   I felt:_____

_____   _____

Snack:_____   I felt:_____

_____   _____

Lunch:_____   I felt:_____

_____   _____

Snack:_____   I felt:_____

_____   _____

Dinner:_____   I felt:_____

_____   _____

Snack:_____   I felt:_____

_____   _____

Glasses of water (8oz) :_____

Other Beverages:_____

Movement for today:_____

Did you take your supplements?   Damn right   I forgot

How was your sleep last night?_____

What was your energy level today?   Low   Eh   Pretty Good   Fan-fucking-tastic!

Today I'm grateful for:

1._____

2._____

3._____

Today is:___ /___ /___

Breakfast:_____   I felt:_____
_____   _____

Snack:_____   I felt:_____
_____   _____

Lunch:_____   I felt:_____
_____   _____

Snack:_____   I felt:_____
_____   _____

Dinner:_____   I felt:_____
_____   _____

Snack:_____   I felt:_____
_____   _____

Glasses of water (8oz) :_____

Other Beverages:_____

Movement for today:_____

Did you take your supplements?   Damn right   I forgot

How was your sleep last night?_____

What was your energy level today?   Low   Eh   Pretty Good   Fan-fucking-tastic!

Today I'm grateful for:

1._____

2._____

3._____

Today is:____ /____ /____

Breakfast:_____   I felt:_____
_____   _____

Snack:_____   I felt:_____
_____   _____

Lunch:_____   I felt:_____
_____   _____

Snack:_____   I felt:_____
_____   _____

Dinner:_____   I felt:_____
_____   _____

Snack:_____   I felt:_____
_____   _____

Glasses of water (8oz) :_____

Other Beverages:_____

Movement for today:_____

Did you take your supplements?   Damn right   I forgot

How was your sleep last night?_____

What was your energy level today?   Low   Eh   Pretty Good   Fan-fucking-tastic!

Today I'm grateful for:

1._____

2._____

3._____

Today is:____ /____ /____

Breakfast:_____   I felt:_____
_____   _____

Snack:_____   I felt:_____
_____   _____

Lunch:_____   I felt:_____
_____   _____

Snack:_____   I felt:_____
_____   _____

Dinner:_____   I felt:_____
_____   _____

Snack:_____   I felt:_____
_____   _____

Glasses of water (8oz) :_____

Other Beverages:_____

Movement for today:_____

Did you take your supplements?   Damn right   I forgot

How was your sleep last night?_____

What was your energy level today?   Low   Eh   Pretty Good   Fan-fucking-tastic!

Today I'm grateful for:

1._____

2._____

3._____

Today is:____ / ____ / ____

Breakfast:_____   I felt:_____

_____   _____

Snack:_____   I felt:_____

_____   _____

Lunch:_____   I felt:_____

_____   _____

Snack:_____   I felt:_____

_____   _____

Dinner:_____   I felt:_____

_____   _____

Snack:_____   I felt:_____

_____   _____

Glasses of water (8oz) :_____

Other Beverages:_____

Movement for today:_____

Did you take your supplements?   Damn right   I forgot

How was your sleep last night?_____

What was your energy level today?   Low   Eh   Pretty Good   Fan-fucking-tastic!

Today I'm grateful for:

1._____

2._____

3._____

Today is:___ /___ /___

Breakfast:_____   I felt:_____
_____   _____

Snack:_____   I felt:_____
_____   _____

Lunch:_____   I felt:_____
_____   _____

Snack:_____   I felt:_____
_____   _____

Dinner:_____   I felt:_____
_____   _____

Snack:_____   I felt:_____
_____   _____

Glasses of water (8oz) :_____

Other Beverages:_____

Movement for today:_____

Did you take your supplements?   Damn right   I forgot

How was your sleep last night?_____

What was your energy level today?   Low   Eh   Pretty Good   Fan-fucking-tastic!

Today I'm grateful for:

1._____

2._____

3._____

Check in, Yo

In general, this week I felt:_____
_____
_____
_____
_____

My self-care practice included:_____
_____
_____
_____
_____

These decisions did not support me:_____
_____
_____
_____
_____

Next week, my goal is:_____
_____
_____
_____
_____

Today is:____ /____ /____

Breakfast:_____   I felt:_____

_____   _____

Snack:_____   I felt:_____

_____   _____

Lunch:_____   I felt:_____

_____   _____

Snack:_____   I felt:_____

_____   _____

Dinner:_____   I felt:_____

_____   _____

Snack:_____   I felt:_____

_____   _____

Glasses of water (8oz) :_____

Other Beverages:_____

Movement for today:_____

Did you take your supplements?   Damn right   I forgot

How was your sleep last night?_____

What was your energy level today?   Low   Eh   Pretty Good   Fan-fucking-tastic!

Today I'm grateful for:

1._____

2._____

3._____

Today is:____ /____ /____

Breakfast:_____   I felt:_____

_____   _____

Snack:_____   I felt:_____

_____   _____

Lunch:_____   I felt:_____

_____   _____

Snack:_____   I felt:_____

_____   _____

Dinner:_____   I felt:_____

_____   _____

Snack:_____   I felt:_____

_____   _____

Glasses of water (8oz) :_____

Other Beverages:_____

Movement for today:_____

Did you take your supplements?   Damn right   I forgot

How was your sleep last night?_____

What was your energy level today?   Low   Eh   Pretty Good   Fan-fucking-tastic!

Today I'm grateful for:

1._____

2._____

3._____

Today is:___ /___ /___

Breakfast:_____   I felt:_____

_____   _____

Snack:_____   I felt:_____

_____   _____

Lunch:_____   I felt:_____

_____   _____

Snack:_____   I felt:_____

_____   _____

Dinner:_____   I felt:_____

_____   _____

Snack:_____   I felt:_____

_____   _____

Glasses of water (8oz) :_____

Other Beverages:_____

Movement for today:_____

Did you take your supplements?   Damn right   I forgot

How was your sleep last night?_____

What was your energy level today?   Low   Eh   Pretty Good   Fan-fucking-tastic!

Today I'm grateful for:

1._____

2._____

3._____

Today is:____ /____ /____

Breakfast:_____ I felt:_____

_____ _____

Snack:_____ I felt:_____

_____ _____

Lunch:_____ I felt:_____

_____ _____

Snack:_____ I felt:_____

_____ _____

Dinner:_____ I felt:_____

_____ _____

Snack:_____ I felt:_____

_____ _____

Glasses of water (8oz) :_____

Other Beverages:_____

Movement for today:_____

Did you take your supplements?   Damn right   I forgot

How was your sleep last night?_____

What was your energy level today?   Low   Eh   Pretty Good   Fan-fucking-tastic!

Today I'm grateful for:

1._____

2._____

3._____

Today is:___ /___ /___

Breakfast:_____   I felt:_____
_____   _____

Snack:_____   I felt:_____
_____   _____

Lunch:_____   I felt:_____
_____   _____

Snack:_____   I felt:_____
_____   _____

Dinner:_____   I felt:_____
_____   _____

Snack:_____   I felt:_____
_____   _____

Glasses of water (8oz) :_____

Other Beverages:_____

Movement for today:_____

Did you take your supplements?   Damn right   I forgot

How was your sleep last night?_____

What was your energy level today? Low   Eh   Pretty Good   Fan-fucking-tastic!

Today I'm grateful for:

1._____

2._____

3._____

Today is:___ /___ /___

Breakfast:_____   I felt:_____
_____   _____

Snack:_____   I felt:_____
_____   _____

Lunch:_____   I felt:_____
_____   _____

Snack:_____   I felt:_____
_____   _____

Dinner:_____   I felt:_____
_____   _____

Snack:_____   I felt:_____
_____   _____

Glasses of water (8oz) :_____

Other Beverages:_____

Movement for today:_____

Did you take your supplements?   Damn right   I forgot

How was your sleep last night?_____

What was your energy level today?   Low   Eh   Pretty Good   Fan-fucking-tastic!

Today I'm grateful for:

1._____

2._____

3._____

Today is:_____ /_____ /_____

Breakfast:_____   I felt:_____
_____   _____

Snack:_____   I felt:_____
_____   _____

Lunch:_____   I felt:_____
_____   _____

Snack:_____   I felt:_____
_____   _____

Dinner:_____   I felt:_____
_____   _____

Snack:_____   I felt:_____
_____   _____

Glasses of water (8oz) :_____

Other Beverages:_____

Movement for today:_____

Did you take your supplements?   Damn right   I forgot

How was your sleep last night?_____

What was your energy level today?   Low   Eh   Pretty Good   Fan-fucking-tastic!

Today I'm grateful for:

1._____

2._____

3._____

Check in, Yo

In general, this week I felt:_____

_____

_____

_____

_____

My self-care practice included:_____

_____

_____

_____

_____

These decisions did not support me:_____

_____

_____

_____

_____

Next week, my goal is:_____

_____

_____

_____

_____

How'd It Go?

Go back through the past month. Do you notice any patterns in your food and mood?

Example: "I felt more tired when I didn't drink water."

"I was happier on days I ate snacks"

"I had more energy when I brought lunch to work"

_____

_____

_____

_____

What are you gonna do about it?

_____

_____

_____

_____

List some awesome things that happened this month:

_____

_____

_____

_____

you fucking deserve everything you desire

Get it.

About Cait Byrnes:

Cait Byrnes is a Holistic Health Coach and Burlesque Performer from the Jersey Shore. Cait earned her Bachelor of Fine Arts from the Maryland Institute College of Art in Baltimore in 2010, and served with the Community Arts Collaborative AmeriCorps program from 2010 to 2013. In 2014, she earned her Certificate in Holistic Health Coaching from the Institute for Integrative Nutrition, and Level 2 Reiki Certification from Reiki Master Andrea Wenger. Cait has worked with several communities in Baltimore to create neighborhood events, parades, and youth programs, and has served as the Assistant Director for the Feminist Art Project - Baltimore Chapter.

Cait believes that womens health is a feminist issue, and that our society teaches girls from a young age that we need to put everyone else's needs before our own.

In her Health Coaching practice, Cait works with women to empower them to put their needs first, and to take their health into their own hands. Her coaching technique includes a mixture of nutrition education, radical self-care, and simple practices for emotional wellness. She works with clients nationwide via phone, and also teaches workshops online and in-person.

Want more health and wellness tips? Check out CaitByrnes.com and get on my mailing list for you weekly dose of badassery.

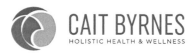

42158613R00060

Made in the USA
Middletown, DE
03 April 2017